Qëndresë Daka
Vladimir Trkulja

Primary Open-Angle Glaucoma Treatment: An Overview of Evidence

Qëndresë Daka
Vladimir Trkulja

Primary Open-Angle Glaucoma Treatment: An Overview of Evidence

LAP LAMBERT Academic Publishing

Impressum / Imprint

Bibliografische Information der Deutschen Nationalbibliothek: Die Deutsche Nationalbibliothek verzeichnet diese Publikation in der Deutschen Nationalbibliografie; detaillierte bibliografische Daten sind im Internet über http://dnb.d-nb.de abrufbar.

Alle in diesem Buch genannten Marken und Produktnamen unterliegen warenzeichen-, marken- oder patentrechtlichem Schutz bzw. sind Warenzeichen oder eingetragene Warenzeichen der jeweiligen Inhaber. Die Wiedergabe von Marken, Produktnamen, Gebrauchsnamen, Handelsnamen, Warenbezeichnungen u.s.w. in diesem Werk berechtigt auch ohne besondere Kennzeichnung nicht zu der Annahme, dass solche Namen im Sinne der Warenzeichen- und Markenschutzgesetzgebung als frei zu betrachten wären und daher von jedermann benutzt werden dürften.

Bibliographic information published by the Deutsche Nationalbibliothek: The Deutsche Nationalbibliothek lists this publication in the Deutsche Nationalbibliografie; detailed bibliographic data are available in the Internet at http://dnb.d-nb.de.

Any brand names and product names mentioned in this book are subject to trademark, brand or patent protection and are trademarks or registered trademarks of their respective holders. The use of brand names, product names, common names, trade names, product descriptions etc. even without a particular marking in this work is in no way to be construed to mean that such names may be regarded as unrestricted in respect of trademark and brand protection legislation and could thus be used by anyone.

Coverbild / Cover image: www.ingimage.com

Verlag / Publisher:
LAP LAMBERT Academic Publishing
ist ein Imprint der / is a trademark of
OmniScriptum GmbH & Co. KG
Heinrich-Böcking-Str. 6-8, 66121 Saarbrücken, Deutschland / Germany
Email: info@lap-publishing.com

Herstellung: siehe letzte Seite /
Printed at: see last page
ISBN: 978-3-659-77423-2

To my lovely family, Dora and Labi,
who are the source of inspiration and encouragement in my life.

Acknowledgements:

I would like to express my highest appreciation to Prof. Vladimir Trkulja for being my mentor and providing me with much needed advice and support. I am deeply thankful to my parents for being my mentors and role models during my whole life.

CONTENTS

ABBREVIATIONS

AAO	American Academy of Ophthalmology
ACG	Angle Closed Glaucoma
AE	Adverse Events
AMSTAR	Assessment of Multiple Systematic Reviews
BET	Betaxolol
BCVA	Best Corrected Visual Acuity
BIMA	Bimatoprost
BRINZ	Brinzolamide
BRIM	Brimonidine
CAIs	Carbonic Anhydrase Inhibitors
CCT	Central Corneal Thickness
C/D Ratio	Cup/Disc Ratio
CHOLINOMIMETICS	Acetylcholine Receptor Agonists
DORZ	Dorzolamide
EGS	European Glaucoma Society
GAT	Goldmann Applanation Tonometry
GON	Glaucoma Optic Neuropathy
GRADE	Grading of Recommendations Assessment, Development and Evaluation
GVFD	Glaucomatous Visual Field Defects
HTG	High Tension Glaucoma
IOP	Intraocular Pressure
LAT	Latanoprost
MeSH	Medical Subject Headings
MYOC	Myocilin Gene
NPTS	Non-Penetrating Trabecular Surgery
NTF4	Neurotrophin 4 Gene
NTG	Normal Tension Glaucoma
NRR	Neuro Retinal Rim
OAG	Open Angle Glaucoma
OBF	Ocular Blood Flow
OCT	Optical Coherence Tomography
OHT	Ocular Hypertension
OHTS	The Ocular Hypertension Treatment Study
ONH	Optic Nerve Head
OPA1	Optic Atrophy 1 Gene
OPTN	Optineurin Gene

PGAs	Prostaglandin Analogues
POAG	Primary Open Angle Glaucoma
PRISMA	Preferred Reporting Items for Systematic review and MetaAnalyses
PT	Publication Type
RCTs	Randomized Controlled Clinical Trials
RGCs	Retinal Ganglion Cells
RNFL	Retinal Nerve Fibre Layer
SLP	Scanning Laser Polarimetry
TB	Trabeculectomy
TIM	Timolol
TRAV	Travoprost
UBM	Ultrasound Biomicroscopy
UC	Unfixed Combinations
UCLT	Unfixed Combination of Latanoprost and Timolol
VF	Visual Field
WDR 36	WD Repeat Domain 36 Gene
WHO	World Health Organization
α-agonists	Alpha-Adrenoceptor Agonists
β-blockers	Beta-Adrenoceptor Antagonists

1. INTRODUCTION

The concept of glaucoma has been refined, especially over the last 100 years, and has evolved from a disease of eye pressure to a disease of optic nerve neuropathy. Currently, glaucoma describes a family of multifactorial optical neuropathies characterized by a progressive loss of retinal ganglion cells (RGCs) leading to a typical optic nerve head (ONH) damage and distinctive visual field (VF) defects (1).

The disease may be manifested with a variety of signs and symptoms, depending upon type and severity, such as: excavation of the optic disk, hardness of the eyeball, corneal anaesthesia, reduced visual acuity, seeing of coloured halos around lights, disturbed dark adaptation, VF defects and headaches. It can lead to blindness in the affected eye if left untreated.

Glaucoma is classified either according to cause, the age of onset, initial pathological event or mechanism. Depending on the presence or absence of ocular or systemic disorders that may contribute to pressure rise, it is classified into primary or secondary glaucoma. It can also be classified into congenital or acquired form. However, the most common, classification into open-angle or angle-closure glaucoma is based on the mechanism by which aqueous outflow is impaired with respect to the anterior chamber angle configuration (Table 1) (2).

Glaucoma remains the leading cause of irreversible blindness worldwide (3-7). It was estimated that by 2010, 79.6 million people around the world would suffer from glaucoma, and of those, 74% with Open Angle Glaucoma (OAG). The total number of patients with OAG in 2020 will be 58.6 million, with the highest number among people of European descent. Population-based studies in developed countries suggest that more than 50% of the prevalent OAG patients are undetected (7), and this estimate is likely to be higher in developing countries (4). Authors of a recent meta-analysis concluded that prevalence of POAG increases more rapidly in Caucasian than in black and Asian populations (8).

Table 1. Classification of primary glaucoma (2).

Open Angle Glaucoma (OAG)	Angle Closure Glaucoma (ACG)	Congenital Glaucoma
Primary Open Angle Glaucoma (POAG)	Primary Angle Closure Suspect	True Congenital
Normal Tension Glaucoma (NTG)	Primary Angle Closure	Infantile Glaucoma
High Tension Glaucoma (HTG)	Primary Angle Closure Glaucoma	Juvenile Glaucoma

1.1. Primary open angle glaucoma (POAG)

There was a lack of consistency in definition of POAG through the years. In different journals, articles from 1980 until now have described the disease differently according to optic disc, VF specifics and IOP criteria (9).

Today, the American Academy of Ophthalmology (AAO) defines POAG as a progressive, chronic optic neuropathy in adults where IOP and other unknown factors contribute to damage. Characteristic acquired atrophy of the optic nerve and loss of RGCs and their axons is not associated with any other identifiable causes. The condition is associated with an anterior chamber angle that is open by gonioscopic appearance (10). IOP is not the key part of the definition and diagnosis is based on the presence of the optic nerve damage, manifested either by optic disc or VF abnormalities. Indeed, the European Glaucoma Society (EGS) definition of POAG has been arbitrarily subdivided into High Tension (HTG) and Normal Tension (NTG) disease according to IOP levels, even though they may represent a spectrum of optic neuropathies variably sensitive to IOP (11).

1.1.1. Primary open angle glaucoma/ High tension glaucoma (HTG)

There is an amount of conflicting literature regarding HTG and NTG. Some studies identified the differences in the appearance of the optic disc and visual field, raising questions of different mechanisms and aetiologies of optic nerve damage in these two clinical entities of POAG. Other studies have found no such relationship, therefore it is difficult to draw any conclusions (12 -14).

Clinically, HTG is characterised by: an excavation of the optic nerve, referred to as glaucomatous optic neuropathy (GON); and glaucomatous visual field defect (GVFD). It is associated with open and normal anterior chamber angle and elevated IOP in absence of any known explanations. The progression of the disease rises continuously with the rise of the IOP level.

1.1.2. Primary open angle glaucoma/ Normal tension glaucoma (NTG)

For many years, occurrence of atrophy and excavation of the ONH in the absence of elevated IOP was considered to be a distinct form of POAG. However, recently, it has been shown that POAG is a continuum disease in which the aetiology extends from being pre dominantly IOP dependent at one end (HTG), to predominantly IOP-independent at the other end (NTG) (15).

It is generally thought that physiological variation of Central Corneal Thickness (CCT) is important only for the IOP measurement but not related to any particular type of POAG. So, related to NTG, it could be that IOP is falsely lower as an error of measurement – that it is actually HTG, but with a thin cornea. Two studies showed that the risk of GON increases by 40% and 30% for every 40 micrometres thinner cornea (16, 17).

Clinically, NTG is characterized by normal IOP without treatment. Except VF defects that in NTG typically appear deeper, steeper and closer to fixation, there are characteristic disc haemorrhages.

1.2. Primary open angle glaucoma suspect

The term POAG suspect is used to define individuals when not all the criteria that define POAG are presented. It refers to an individual with clinical findings or risk factors that indicate an increased likelihood of developing POAG.

Clinically, POAG suspects may have one of the clinical findings in at least one eye with open anterior chamber: appearance of the ONH or retinal nerve fibre layer (RNFL) that is suspicious for glaucomatous damage; a VF suspicious for glaucomatous damage in the absence of clinical signs of other optic neuropathies; or consistently elevated IOP associated with normal appearance of the ONH and RNFL and with normal VF test results. The definition excludes known secondary causes for OAG (11, 18).

1.3. Ocular hypertension (OHT)

Over the years, the word "*preglaucoma*" was used to define individuals with an elevated IOP and without detectable glaucomatous damage in the standard clinical eye and VF examination, although the majority of them never developed POAG (19).

Diagnosis between ocular hypertension (OHT) and early POAG is often difficult. In a review published in 1998, authors found that 20% of the papers published in the last 15 years used raised IOP as the only criteria to diagnose glaucoma (20).

Today, the OHT term is widely used for research and classification purposes for individuals with IOP higher than 21 mmHg but without any VF, ONH and RNFL changes. EGS in its classification states, that the term OHT should only be used to indicate that the IOP is consistently outside two or three standard deviations from the normal mean, with all other ocular findings within normal limits (11).

1.2. Etiology

The exact etiology of the POAG remains unknown and still relatively poorly understood despite numerous research in this area. Furthermore, for many years, authors have suggested that HTG and NTG represent clinical entities with different pathogenesis and risk factor implications.

According to data from newer studies, NTG and HTG represent a continuum disease in which elevated IOP is the predominant risk factor, while additional independent factors take increasing importance in NTG (21).

1.2.1. Risk factors

From the risk factors that may influence POAG, IOP is the most studied. IOP is causal and changeable, and is the main clinically treatable risk factor that can help prevent POAG (22).

In humans, IOP has a non-Gaussian distribution with a mean of 16 mmHg and two standard deviations on either side that gives a range of normal IOP from 11-21mmHg. Although, many eyes with IOP above the average range do not develop glaucoma and others within normal range of IOP develop it, it is noticed that, the higher the IOP, the greater the likelihood of glaucoma. In addition to the level of IOP, it seems that of relevance is also circadian and day to day IOP fluctuation (23, 24).

Several other ocular, systemic and general risk factors have been proposed to play a role in the POAG pathogenesis and conversion of OHT to POAG but the most studied and with the growing body of evidence are: age, race, ethnicity, family history, genetics, vascular factors, diabetes mellitus, myopia, corneal thickness, and ONH (Table 2). Some books also mention lifestyle, socioeconomic status, alcohol consumption or smoking as possible risk factors.

Table 2. Risk factors that may contribute in POAG development.

AGE	Prevalence studies demonstrate that it is unusual to see the disease before the age of 40, and more than three times higher after the age of 65. It is believed that damage progresses faster in older people.	2, 19, 22
RACE	Prevalence studies state that POAG prevalence in black people is higher, develops earlier and is more severe, while NTG occurs more in Japan.	2, 10
FAMILY HISTORY	Responsible genes can show incomplete penetrance and variable expressivity in some families. IOP, facility of aqueous outflow and optic disc size are also genetically determined. First-degree relatives of patients with POAG are at an increased risk.	2, 10, 19
GENETICS	Genetic studies detected different mutation in loci of the human genome associated with POAG like: *MYOC, OPTN, WDR36, OPA1* and the *NTF*.	10, 22
GENDER	Studies did not find a clear-cut evidence of gender as a risk factor, although some studies have found a higher prevalence of NTG in females.	2, 22
ONH	For many years enlarged ONH was considered as a risk factor. Recently, cup/disc ratio, cup/disc ratio asymmetry and pattern standard deviation are described as additional risk factors.	24, 25
CCT	CCT is lower in NTG patients and higher in people with OHT. Indeed, CCT, curvature of the cornea, and cornea biomechanics can all affect the measurement of IOP.	24, 25
MYOPIA	It is thought that myopic eyes maybe at increased risk for POAG. However, people with myopia are more likely to seek eye care and thus have a higher probability of having glaucoma detected early.	10, 19, 22
VASCULAR DISEASES	The higher probability of involvement of vascular factors is when POAG occurs/progresses at lower IOPs. A range of vascular diseases is thought to be associated with the development and progression of the disease.	19, 24
DIABETES MELLITUS	There are some studies that show a correlation between diabetes mellitus and POAG, but it still remains controversial if diabetes is an independent risk factor.	2, 19

POAG = Primary Open Angle Glaucoma; NTG = Normal Tension Glaucoma; IOP = Intraocular Pressure; *MYOC* = Myocilin; *OPTN* = Optineurin; *NTF4* = Neurotrophin; 4; *WDR36* = WD Repeat Domain 36; *OPA1*= Optic Atrophy 1. ONH = Optic Nerve Heat; OHT=Ocular Hypertension; CCT = Central Corneal Thickness.

1.2.2. Pathophysiology

A definitive description of the pathophysiological processes that cause characteristic atrophy of the optic nerve and loss of RGCs in POAG still needs to be established. In POAG, RGC death occurs predominantly through apoptosis rather than necrosis. Loss of axons, blood vessels and glial cells cause tissue remodelling, leading to the enlargement or the asymmetrical deep of the optic cup, optic disc haemorrhage, peripapillary atrophy, neuroretinal rim (NRR) and RNFL thinning that are unique for GON (26, 27). Several theories have been suggested to describe the occurrence of optic neuropathy in POAG. Most widely studied are the mechanical and vascular theory, but it is generally recognized that POAG can be caused by a mixture of both mechanisms.

The mechanical theory is based on the mechanical force that causes elevated IOP in lamina cribrosa, glia and axons of ONH. In the context of mechanical theory, it is believed that pressure gradient around the ONH is more important rather than the absolute IOP. According to this theory, direct compression of axons and the deformation of the pores and channels of the lamina cribrosa disrupts axoplasmic flow and leads to RGCs death (28). However, affection of ONH in NTG beside the normal IOP level, and absence of GON in OHT despite the elevated IOP leads to idea that in individuals alternative or additional causative factors contribute to the development of GON.

The vascular theory is based on the ischemic and hypoxic insult of the ONH tissues due to instability of blood flow in the microvasculature that supplies ONH (29, 30). Possible mechanisms may extend from: losing of capillaries, reductions in blood flow, failure of vascular regulation, interference with delivery of nutrients or removal of metabolic products from axons, and increases in vessel rigidity at both levels (2, 24). A lot of research has been conducted to explore the role of ocular and systemic vascular factors in the pathophysiology of POAG, but still they are not well understood and remain controversial.

1.3. Diagnosis

For the proper management of POAG, comprehensive evaluation of the eye is important. It can reveal the diagnosis, severity, and progression of the disease. All components of the eye evaluation should be performed and more than one visit is required (10, 31). Identification of POAG may require a variety of modalities for the clinical examination, but some are particularly important.

1.3.1. Anamnesis

POAG has a painless and insidious nature, therefore patients usually do not report symptoms during the early phase. Very rarely, patients with will note brow arch and haloes around lights. Visual acuity alternation occurs only in advanced disease or when *scotoma* is close to fixation, and VF defects are not consciously perceived by patients (24, 32). Some patients may suffer from loss of chromatic or achromatic sensitivity, reduced contrast sensitivity, and increased blur.

The initial examination history should include: ocular, family, and systemic risk factors history. An assessment of the impact of patient's visual function in relation to hobbies, employment, and daily living should be performed (23).

1.3.2. Clinical examination

Evaluation of the refraction should be done to obtain the best corrected visual acuity (BCVA) that is crucial for accurate VF testing, but also to exclude clinical confusion of disc morphologies that can be due to early myopia (19). Pupils should be examined for reactivity and afferent pupil defect that may be present in eyes with advanced optic nerve damage in highly asymmetric cases of POAG. Examination of the anterior segment in slit-lamp should be done to exclude other forms of glaucoma or ocular pathologies.

1.3.3. Tonometry

Tonometry should always be performed before gonioscopy and pupil dilatation. Beside for diagnosis, tonometry is also important for evaluation of the treatment effect. Since IOP can be fluctuated by the influence of numerous factors like: time of day, heartbeat, respiration, exercise, fluid intake, topical and systemic medications, tonometry should be recorded at different hours of the day or on different days (19). This way of measurement is important to: establish the diagnosis of NTG, stop the progression of POAG due to unrecognized fluctuations, and evaluate the ability of anti-glaucoma therapies to lower the IOP throughout the 24h day (33-35). A number of tonometers utilizing different techniques have been produced. Goldman Applanation Tonometer (GAT) remains the preferred one and relatively accurate, whereas non-contact tonometers used more for screening purposes are less precise.

1.3.4. Pachymetry

Measurement of CCT is recommended as it influences GAT readings. However, there is no agreement as to whether there is a validated correction algorithm for GAT and CCT (20, 36). Normal CCT is 540+/-30μm, whereas each glaucoma cabinet has tables for correction of IOP in respect to pachymetry findings.

1.3.5. Corneal hysteresis

Corneal hysteresis (CH) measurement is recommended as it reflects the viscoelastic properties of the cornea. CH does not show any significant variations throughout the day (22), and has greater impact than CCT and corneal curvature in the IOP measurement errors (37). Low CH value is a risk factor for underestimation of the IOP and a high CH value for overestimation, however, CCT and CH are independently associated with IOP (38).

1.3.6. Gonioscopy

POAG diagnosis requires careful evaluation of the anterior chamber angle in order to exclude secondary causes of IOP elevation. Either indirect or direct gonioscopy techniques can be performed for this purpose (39). Beyond gonioscopy, that is a subjective technique, imaging techniques for evaluation of the anterior chamber angle are: ultrasound biomicroscopy (UBM) and anterior segment optical coherence tomography (OCT). These two techniques are non-invasive, but do not replace the goniosocpy and are used just as complements (22).

1.3.7. Optic nerve head and retinal nerve fibre layer examination

In POAG diagnosis and management the most critical part is evaluation of ONH and RNFL. Alternations in ONH and RNFL are the most typical signs of POAG, and often occur before VF defects (28). Relevant variables that can be noticed are: NRR thickness, disc asymmetry, pallor of the disc, disc haemorrhages, peripapillary atrophy, blood vessel changes, visibility and loss of RNFL. These data should be collected in drawings, whereas quantitative measurements by instruments should be performed. Evaluation techniques for these structures involve: subjective techniques (ophthalmoscopy), stereoscopic fundus photography and imaging techniques. The most common used imaging techniques are: scanning laser polarimetry (SLP), confocal scanning laser tomography (CSLT), time domain and spectral domain OCT.

1.3.8. Visual Field Function

Except ONH and RNFL evaluation, VF test is crucial for POAG diagnosing and management. This psychophysical test remains the primary visual function test performed as it reflects characteristic changes of the RNFL anatomy, and determines the impact of VF on a patient's quality of life and activities of daily living (40, 41). Currently, the most preferable technique for VF assessment is the automated static perimtery. Suprathreshold static perimetry is suited for rapid screening, while manual perimetry remains helpful in documenting defects outside the central 30° and in monitoring end-stage VF loss (10). Sensitive assessment of POAG progression can be performed by independent programs that calculate and compare VFs (42).

1.3.9. Electrophysiology

Electrophysiological examination techniques provide localised information of RGCs function. In POAG, RCGs are lost before the appearance of subjective VF defects (43), however, electroretinography and visually evoked potentials examinations are not routinely performed due to the long-time of performing. They are a part of the objective testing when patients are not able to perform perimetry.

1.3.10. Genetic Testing

Genetic tests for POAG are still not routinely performed, although they may be helpful to screen individuals in risk and decide for therapy. Association of the genes with POAG does not have the specificity required for a gene-based diagnostic or screening test. Furthermore, they can be carried out only in specialised laboratories.

1.3.11. Ocular Blood Flow Measurement

Indications for the measurement of ocular blood flow (OBF) are based on the possible influence of vascular risk factors in the POAG disease. The assessment is not supported by evidence, and the ideal test to measure comprehensive OBF of patients is yet to be developed. Furthermore, information is practically useless for clinicians, whereas only few guidelines recommend treatment of POAG patients in regard to reduced OBF (44).

1.4. Treatment

The aim of therapy in POAG is to prevent functional impairment of vision by slowing down the apoptosis of RGCs within a patient's lifetime. This aim reveals many questions: when should the treatment start, who should be treated and how he should be treated. Therefore, POAG treatment requires strong collaboration with patients.

Elevated IOP, which is the main factor implicated in the mechanisms that are thought to precipitate RCGs apoptosis in POAG, is currently the only treatable factor approved by many guidelines (10, 11). Studies demonstrated that decreasing of IOP prevented both conversion of OHT to POAG and progression of POAG (45, 46). The treatment modalities for elevated IOP include: medical, laser, surgical or combined therapy, but it is questionable which modality of the IOP-lowering therapy is the most effective, with the fewest adverse effects and lowest cost.

Non-IOP lowering treatment modalities toward factors that may play a role in POAG pathogenesis are being investigated (47, 48), but until now neither showed enough evidence.

1.4.1. Medical therapy

Medical therapy has an important role in POAG treatment, especially in the last years that the pharmaceutical market has presented a variety of topical IOP lowering drugs. These drugs are considered as the first line of treatment, and in most patients they can control the disease alone. Patient compliance is very important for this type of treatment, their adherence and persistence to the therapy is a key of successful management.

Topical IOP lowering drugs reduce elevated IOP either by reducing aqueous production or by increasing aqueous outflow through the conventional or the unconventional pathway (49).They are formulated as aqueous solutions, suspensions, ointments, inserts, emulsions, and gels. Table 3 summarizes five major classes of IOP-lowering drugs: direct and indirect acetylcholine receptor agonists (cholinomimetics); alpha-adrenoceptor agonists (α-agonists); carbonic anhydrase inhibitors (CAIs); beta-adrenoceptor antagonists (β-blockers); and prostaglandin analogues (PGAs) (50, 51). Each group comprises of several individual drugs, whereas fixed combinations are also available. Some drugs are not used anymore as the new drugs from the same group which have greater effect and less adverse effects became available.

Table 3. Five major classes of IOP-lowering drugs.

α-agonists	β-blockers	CAIs	PGAs	Cholinomimetics
Dipivefrin	Timolol	Acetazolamide	Travaprost	Pilocarpine
Brimonidine	Levobunolol	Methazolamide	Latanaprost	Carbachol
Apraclonidine	Betaxolol	Dorzolamide	Brimatoprost	Physostigmine
Epinephrine	Carteolol	Brinzolamide	Tafluprost	Echothiopate
Clonidine	Metipranolol	Diclorphenamide	Unoprostone	Demecarium
	Pindolol			Aceclidine
	Befunolol			Achetylcoline

α-agonists = Alpha-Adrenoreceptor Agonists; β-blockers = Beta-Adrenoreceptor Antagonists;
CAIs = Carbonic Anhydrase Inhibitors; PGAs = Prostaglandin Analogues;
Cholinomimetics = Direct and Indirect Acetylcholine Receptor Agonists.

1.4.2. Laser therapy

In POAG treatment, at first, laser therapy was considered only when medical therapy failed. Lasers were used mainly before surgical procedures that could cause adverse effects including bleb-associated problems, cataracts, and infections (17). Today, they can be considered as a first line therapy in some patients, usually adjunct to medical therapy or with attempt to gradually withdraw medical therapy (19). Even so, the reduction of medication is a secondary consideration.

Laser procedures used to lower IOP include: trabeculoplasty, iridotomy, iridoplasty and cycloablation. Laser trabeculoplasty is a procedure most commonly used in the case of POAG. It lowers IOP by targeting trabecular meshwork by argon diode and selective laser or alternative lasers like: continuous wave length lasers of red and infrared wavelengths (24).

1.4.3. Surgical therapy

Indications for IOP lowering surgical procedures in POAG patients changed since the introduction of novel surgery devices with low morbidity for surgical intervention. Still, they remain the second line of treatment. In POAG patients, surgery is considered only when maximal drug therapy is not effective, although it can reduce the number of patient visits to the doctor.

Commonly performed surgery is a partial thickness procedure called guarded trabeculectomy, its goal is to create a new pathway for the flow of aqueous humour from the anterior chamber in to the subconjunctival and sub-Tenon spaces. To prevent failure of filtration, several modifications of this procedure evolved with the use of anti-metabolites agents and aqueous shunts (11, 19). Recently, several non-penetrating surgeries that avoid a continuous passageway from the anterior chamber to the subconjunctival space have been presented. The two main types are viscocanalostomy and non-penetrating deep sclerectomy.

The newest aim of the IOP lowering surgery is to enhance the physiologic outflow of the eye by passive filtration of the humour aqueous in the trabecular outflow. These novel surgical approaches include: trabecular stent, removing of an arc of trabecular meshwork and inner wall of Schlemm's via electro-ablation with simultaneous infusion of fluid and aspiration of tissue debris (28). These options are not so studied and require special skills and instruments (23, 52). Combined surgeries for POAG and cataracts are lately often performed as prevalence of both diseases increases with age (22, 53).

1.5. Public health consequences

In POAG the destruction of the optical nerve is usually slow and VF loss starts normally in the peripheral vision, therefore many affected individuals are unaware of the disease. Late detection with a consequent delayed treatment commencement is a major risk factor for blindness as visual loss cannot be reversed. However, if diagnosed and treated in time, most POAG patients will retain useful vision for their entire lives.

It was estimated that 20 years after the diagnosis and treatment of POAG, incidence of blindness was 27% unilateral and 9% bilateral (54). Many issues related to blindness are linked to poverty, therefore, incidence of blindness maybe higher in developing countries where the diagnosis and treatment of the disease are delayed. In these countries, visual loss from POAG is especially problematic due to their limited public health resources for diagnosis, treatment and reimbursement of POAG patients.

In many parts of the world, sophistication and efficacy of POAG diagnostic and therapeutic methods rely on expensive equipment and drugs, while research is focused in etiological issues. In developing countries, the primary goal is adequate preventive and therapeutic care of the disease related to their limited budget (55). To achieve this aim, these countries have to approve a public health strategy for POAG treatment with the lowest-cost intervention. Although the economic evaluation of POAG is in its infancy, practical adaptation of data analysis for treatment modalities is highly important for these countries, because physicians and regulations often adopt non cost-effective strategies enhancing the perception of findings (55, 56).

2. EVIDENCE ON POAG TREATMENT

As illustrated already by its classification, glaucoma in general is a very complex and multifaceted condition, whereas POAG is by far more prevalent and bears the major part of the overall healthcare burden of glaucoma.

Although not without controversy, the definition and clinical characteristics of POAG are well defined, but the primary cause that triggers the cascade of events resulting in POAG is less clear. Results from recent studies suggest that, beside elevated IOP, there are other factors that may play a role in the POAG pathogenesis. Treatment modalities towards these factors are being investigated, but still, IOP lowering treatment is the only modality approved for prevention and treatment of the disease.

Management of elevated IOP in OHT individual and POAG patients with IOP-lowering treatment starts initially with topical pharmacological therapy, whereas laser and surgical options are implemented mainly when conservative therapy is not effective, not tolerated or not utilized by the patient (57). Guidelines recommend to reduce IOP by 20-30% from the baseline and to start treatment with a first-line treatment (10,11). If the first-line treatment is not effective, it can be substituted or combined with other compounds (57). Beside efficacy, a rational first line POAG treatment should aim for the fewest side-effects and high cost-effective profile.

A recent overview (57) demonstrated that the number of primary studies and systematic reviews that address POAG has been increased extremely over the past few years due to continuous research inters in this topic. Evaluation of the evidence that is related to relative efficacy, safety and cost-effectiveness profile of IOP lowering treatments for POAG is warranted to improve the public health strategies for coping with the overall burden of the disease. Under such circumstances, a systematic synthesis of the existing evidence appears to be an appropriate methodological approach to achieve the aim of improved overall treatment of POAG. In the context of evidence-based medicine, systematic reviews/meta-analyses are generally considered to provide the highest level of evidence based on filtered data.

With the aim to derive the best evidence on POAG treatment, the present study was conceived as an overview of systematic reviews: a method of identification; qualitative and quantitative evaluation; and synthesis of the available clinical evidence about the posed research questions. In this respect, the present overview aimed to answer specific questions on POAG treatment that could be helpful for the improvement of the public health strategies:

- What is the existing evidence on relative efficacy of IOP-lowering treatments for POAG?

- What is the existing evidence on relative safety of IOP-lowering treatments for POAG?

- What is the existing evidence on cost-effectiveness profile of the IOP-lowering interventions in the treatment of POAG?

3. METHODOLOGY

The present overview followed the format and methods for an overview of systematic reviews as proposed by the current Cochrane Handbook for Systematic Reviews (58). The common methodological elements include: literature search; selection of studies; data collection; assessment of study quality; data synthesis; and evaluation of the quality of evidence.

Most of the methodological characteristics are common to all overviews of reviews. However, an overview of reviews has certain methodological features that depend on whether it deals with epidemiologic, therapeutic or economic issues of the disease. This section depicts the common methodological characteristics of the overview, followed by the methodological particulars for the included systematic reviews for each posed question.

3.1. Literature search

All performed literature searches included searches of electronic databases of published studies, as well as reference lists of identified relevant publications.

Common search strategy was predefined, whereas direct search terms and control terms were adapted to each database. Assistance of a professional librarian was used in this step. All searches were conceived to be sensitive not specific, hence no restrictions were set in respect to the journal, publication date, geographical location or language.

PUBMED, COCHRANE and SCOPUS electronic databases were searched for potential relevant studies during 2014. Search terms used were: "systematic review", "meta-analysis", "review" to identify the study design; "glaucoma", "open angle glaucoma" to identify the condition; and "management", "therapy", "treatment", "intervention", "cost-effective" etc to identify intervention. Protocol for search strategy is depicted in Table 4.

Table 4. Search strategy for systematic reviews/meta-analyses on POAG treatment.

1. Meta-analysis [pt]	37. Unoprostone [All fields, MeSH terms]
2. Meta-analysis [All Fields]	38. Tafluprost [All fields, MeSH terms]
3 Systematic review [pt]	39. Adrenergic alpha-agonists [All fields]
4. Systematic review [All Fields]	40. Apraclonidine [All fields, MeSH terms]
5. Review [pt]	41. Brimonidine [All fields, MeSH terms]
6. Review[All Fields]	42. Epinephrine [All fields, MeSH terms]
7. 1 OR 6	43. Dipivefrin [All fields, MeSH terms]
8. POAG [All fields]	44. Clonidine [All fields, MeSH terms]
9. Primary open angle glaucoma [All Fields]	45. Cholinomimetics [MeSH terms]
10. Open angle glaucoma [All Fields]	46. Pilocarpine [All fields, MeSH terms]
11. Open angle [All Fields]	47. Carbachol [All fields, MeSH terms]
12. Glaucoma [All Fields]	48. Physostigmine [All fields, MeSH terms]
13. Glaucoma, open angle [MeSH Terms]	49. Echothiophate [All fields, MeSH terms]
14. Normal Tension Glaucoma [All Fields]	50. Demecarium [All fields, MeSH terms]
15. Normal Pressure Glaucoma[All Fields]	51. Aceclidine [All fields, MeSH terms]
16. High Tension Glaucoma[All Fields]	52. Acetylcholine [All fields, MeSH terms]
17. High Pressure Glaucoma[All Fields]	53. Carbonic Anhydrase Inhibitors [All fields]
18. 8 OR 17	54. Acetazolamide [All fields, MeSH terms]
19. 7 AND 18	55. Brinzolamide [All fields, MeSH terms]
20. Management[All Fields]	56. Dorzolamide [All fields, MeSH terms]
21. Intervention[All Fields]	57. Dichlorphenamide [All fields]
22. Treatment[All Fields]	58. Methazolamide [All fields, MeSH terms]
23. Prevention[All Fields]	59. Tafluprost [All fields, MeSH terms]
24. Therapy[All Fields]	60. Laser [All Fields]
25. Drug [All Fields]	61. Trabeculoplasty
26. Befunolol [All fields, MeSH Terms]	62. Iridotomy
27. Timolol [All field, MeSH terms]	63. Iridoplasty
28. Metipranolol [All fields, MeSH terms]	64. Cycloablation
29. Carteolol [All fields, MeSH terms]	65. Surgery[All Fields]
30. Levobunolol [All fields, MeSH terms]	66. Trabeculectomy
31. Betaxolol [All fields, MeSH Terms]	67. Viscocanalostomy
32. Pindolol [All fields, MeSH terms]	68. Sclerectomy
33. Prostanglandins, Synthetic [All fields]	69. Effectiveness [All Fields]
34. Latanoprost [All fields, MeSH terms]	70. Cost-effectiveness [All Fields]
35. Travoprost [All fields, MeSH terms]	71. 20 OR 70
36. Bimatoprost [All fields, MeSH terms]	72. 19 AND 71

MeSH = Medical Subject Headings; pt = Publication Type.

3.2. Selection of studies

The inclusion of systematic reviews/meta-analysis in the present overview was based on predefined criteria. The entire process consisted of the following steps:

I. Identification and removal of duplicate publications from the records identified by the initial search;

II. Screening of non-duplicates based on titles and abstracts for potential eligibility for inclusion;

III. Retrieval and full text evaluation of the selected studies for final assessment of eligibility for inclusion.

To be included in the overview, studies had to meet the following criteria:

a. be either systematic reviews or meta-analyses embracing high quality primary studies;

b. include at least 85% POAG patients (as defined by AAO) in individual trials, or across all included primary trial. Both HTG and NTG patients were considered since there is no clear distinction between the two conditions apart from the values of IOP; individuals with ocular hypertension (OHT) were also considered as they are usually treated to prevent POAG development.

c. assess any therapeutic intervention;

d. evaluate either efficacy (IOP, VF, ONH); safety (incidence of adverse events or withdrawals due to adverse events): or cost-effectiveness profile (individual treatments or comparative evaluations) of interventions.

In the overview are not included following studies:

a. individual studies;

b. narrative reviews and reviews reported only in the abstract form;

c. reviews dealing with secondary OAG or ACG.

3.3. Data collection

Data collection forms were previously defined in the protocol. Table 5 depicts main characteristics that had to be extracted in data collection forms. They were designed in order to collect:

I. Descriptive data on included systematic reviews/meta-analyses;

II. Data relevant for quality assessment of included systematic reviews/meta-analyses;

III. Data of the effect measures provided by systematic reviews/meta-analyses.

Table 5. Data collection form for systematic reviews or meta-analyses.

REFERENCE NUMBER:					
REFERENCE TITLE:					
Descriptive Data		**Relevant data for quality assessment**		**Data of the effect measures**	
Author name		Reporting of background		Results of primary outcome	
Publication year		Reporting of methodology		Results of secondary outcomes	
The number and type of included studies		Reporting of results		Limitations of study's methods/results	
Number of patients		Reporting of discussion		Scientific quality	
Evaluated questions		Reporting of conclusion		Key conclusions of study authors	
Outcomes Measured		Reporting of conflicts of interest			

3.4. Assessment of methodological quality

Included systematic reviews/meta-analyses were assessed for both reporting and technical quality, and then were graded for their methodological quality. These elements were assessed using validated tools.

I. PRISMA checklist (59) was used to assess reporting quality of the systematic reviews/meta-analysis. This checklist is not a quality assessment instrument to gauge the methodological quality of a systematic review. The checklist is designed to meet the needs characteristic for reporting of systematic reviews/meta-analyses of randomized controlled trials (RCTs), but it can be used as a basis for reporting of systematic reviews/meta-analysis of other types of research, particularly evaluations of interventions. It includes items that are common to any systematic review/meta-analysis, but also items typical for the RCT methodology: e.g., blinding, randomization, allocation concealment, intention-to-treat (ITT) analysis. PRSIMA checklist is depicted in Table 6 (59).

II. Cochrane Handbook for Systematic Reviews (58) was consulted to evaluate quality of methods used in systematic reviews/meta-analysis to assess: the level of various biases in primary studies; methods to protect from the publication bias; methods undertaken at the systematic review level to reduce biases arising from individual studies; and data pooling techniques.

III. AMSTAR tool (60) was used to assign the methodological quality score of systematic reviews/meta-analyses. AMSTAR is a validated tool (60) for grading the methodological quality of systematic reviews, regardless whether they deal with observational or interventional primary studies. However, it does not categorize them by quality: simply, 1 is the lowest and 11 is the highest level of quality of an individual review (61). AMSTAR tool is depicted in Table 7 (60).

Table 6. The PRISMA checklist for evaluation and reporting of meta-analysis of interventional studies (59).

Section/topic	Item No	Checklist item	Reported on page No
Title			
Title	1	Identify the report as a systematic review, meta-analysis, or both	
Abstract			
Structured summary	2	Provide a structured summary including, as applicable, background, objectives, data sources, study eligibility criteria, participants, interventions, study appraisal and synthesis methods, results, limitations, conclusions and implications of key findings, systematic review registration number	
Introduction			
Rationale	3	Describe the rationale for the review in the context of what is already known	
Objectives	4	Provide an explicit statement of questions being addressed with reference to participants, interventions, comparisons, outcomes, and study design (PICOS)	
Methods			
Protocol and registration	5	Indicate if a review protocol exists, if and where it can be accessed (such as web address), and, if available, provide registration information including registration number	
Eligibility criteria	6	Specify study characteristics (such as PICOS, length of follow-up) and report characteristics (such as years considered, language, publication status) used as criteria for eligibility, giving rationale	
Information sources	7	Describe all information sources (such as databases with dates of coverage, contact with study authors to identify additional studies) in the search and date last searched	
Search	8	Present full electronic search strategy for at least one database, including any limits used, such that it could be repeated	
Study selection	9	State the process for selecting studies (that is, screening, eligibility, included in systematic review, and, if applicable, included in the meta-analysis)	
Data collection process	10	Describe method of data extraction from reports (such as piloted forms, independently, in duplicate) and any processes for obtaining and confirming data from investigators	
Data items	11	List and define all variables for which data were sought (such as PICOS, funding sources) and any assumptions and simplifications made	
Risk of bias in individual studies	12	Describe methods used for assessing risk of bias of individual studies (including specification of whether this was done at the study or outcome level), and how this information is to be used in any data synthesis	
Summary measures	13	State the principal summary measures (such as risk ratio, difference in means).	

Section/topic	Item No	Checklist item	Reported on page No
Synthesis of results	14	Describe the methods of handling data and combining results of studies, if done, including measures of consistency (such as I^2 statistic) for each meta-analysis	
Risk of bias across studies	15	Specify any assessment of risk of bias that may affect the cumulative evidence (such as publication bias, selective reporting within studies)	
Additional analyses	16	Describe methods of additional analyses (such as sensitivity or subgroup analyses, meta-regression), if done, indicating which were pre-specified	
Results			
Study selection	17	Give numbers of studies screened, assessed for eligibility, and included in the review, with reasons for exclusions at each stage, ideally with a flow diagram	
Study characteristics	18	For each study, present characteristics for which data were extracted (such as study size, PICOS, follow-up period) and provide the citations	
Risk of bias within studies	19	Present data on risk of bias of each study and, if available, any outcome-level assessment (see item 12).	
Results of individual studies	20	For all outcomes considered (benefits or harms), present for each study (a) simple summary data for each intervention group and (b) effect estimates and confidence intervals, ideally with a forest plot	
Synthesis of results	21	Present results of each meta-analysis done, including confidence intervals and measures of consistency	
Risk of bias across studies	22	Present results of any assessment of risk of bias across studies (see item 15)	
Additional analysis	23	Give results of additional analyses, if done (such as sensitivity or subgroup analyses, meta-regression) (see item 16)	
Discussion			
Summary of evidence	24	Summarise the main findings including the strength of evidence for each main outcome; consider their relevance to key groups (such as health care providers, users, and policy makers)	
Limitations	25	Discuss limitations at study and outcome level (such as risk of bias), and at review level (such as incomplete retrieval of identified research, reporting bias)	
Conclusions	26	Provide a general interpretation of the results in the context of other evidence, and implications for future research	
Funding			
Funding	27	Describe sources of funding for the systematic review and other support (such as supply of data) and role of funders for the systematic review	

Table 7. The AMSTAR tool for assessing the methodological quality of systematic reviews (60).

1. Was an 'a priori' design provided? The research question and inclusion criteria should be established before the conduct of the review.	☐ Yes ☐ No ☐ Can't answer ☐ Not applicable
2. Was there duplicate study selection and data extraction? There should be at least two independent data extractors and a consensus procedure for disagreements should be in place.	☐ Yes ☐ No ☐ Can't answer ☐ Not applicable
3. Was a comprehensive literature search performed? At least two electronic sources should be searched. The report must include years and databases used (e.g. Central, EMBASE, and MEDLINE). Key words and/or MESH terms must be stated and where feasible the search strategy should be provided. All searches should be supplemented by consulting current contents, reviews, textbooks, specialized registers, or experts in the particular field of study, and by reviewing the references in the studies found.	☐ Yes ☐ No ☐ Can't answer ☐ Not applicable
4. Was the status of publication (i.e. grey literature) used as an inclusion criterion? The authors should state that they searched for reports regardless of their publication type. The authors should state whether or not they excluded any reports (from the systematic review), based on their publication status, language etc.	☐ Yes ☐ No ☐ Can't answer ☐ Not applicable
5. Was a list of studies (included and excluded) provided? A list of included and excluded studies should be provided.	☐ Yes ☐ No ☐ Can't answer ☐ Not applicable
6. Were the characteristics of the included studies provided? In an aggregated form such as a table, data from the original studies should be provided on the participants, interventions and outcomes. The ranges of characteristics in all the studies analyzed e.g. age, race, sex, relevant socioeconomic data, disease status, duration, severity, or other diseases should be reported.	☐ Yes ☐ No ☐ Can't answer ☐ Not applicable
7. Was the scientific quality of the included studies assessed and documented? 'A priori' methods of assessment should be provided (e.g., for effectiveness studies if the author(s) chose to include only randomized, double-blind, placebo controlled studies, or allocation concealment as inclusion criteria); for other types of studies alternative items will be relevant.	☐ Yes ☐ No ☐ Can't answer ☐ Not applicable
8. Was the scientific quality of the included studies used appropriately in formulating conclusions? The results of the methodological rigor and scientific quality should be considered in the analysis and the conclusions of the review, and explicitly stated in formulating recommendations.	☐ Yes ☐ No ☐ Can't answer ☐ Not applicable
9. Were the methods used to combine the findings of studies appropriate? For the pooled results, a test should be done to ensure the studies were combinable, to assess their homogeneity (i.e. Chi-squared test for homogeneity, I^2). If heterogeneity exists a random effects model should be used and/or the clinical appropriateness of combining should be taken into consideration (i.e. is it sensible to combine?).	☐ Yes ☐ No ☐ Can't answer ☐ Not applicable
10. Was the likelihood of publication bias assessed? An assessment of publication bias should include a combination of graphical aids (e.g., funnel plot, other available tests) and/or statistical tests (e.g., Egger regression test).	☐ Yes ☐ No ☐ Can't answer ☐ Not applicable
11. Was the conflict of interest stated? Potential sources of support should be clearly acknowledged in both the systematic review and the included studies.	☐ Yes ☐ No ☐ Can't answer ☐ Not applicable

3.5. Data synthesis/Quality of evidence

Finally, data from the total body of evidence were synthesized as recommended by the Cochrane Handbook (58). All relevant systematic reviews/meta-analyses were evaluated for the quality of the evidence and graded by the GRADE system (62), those that attained at least "moderate quality" level were used to derive answers to the posed research questions.

The GRADE system (63 - 71) is a complex and a comprehensive approach of assessing quality of evidence in healthcare that can be applied to either individual studies or systematic reviews/meta-analyses. This system goes beyond what is assessed by the AMSTAR tool. The GRADE system does not consider only the methodological quality, but also technical correctness. To reach the final grade, it evaluates 5 domains: indirectness, limitations/bias, inconsistency, imprecision and publication bias.

The process of grading starts with an "a priori" grade that could either be reduced or increased. It assigns one of the 4 categories of "quality" to the "body of evidence", as depicted in Table 8. According to GRADE system, evidence from systematic reviews/meta-analyses has a "high quality" starting point. Each of the above 5 domains is assessed and the starting grade is either unchanged, or reduced by 1 or 2 steps. Theoretically, they could also be upgraded by the presented criteria.

Table 8. The GRADE system categorization of "quality of the body of evidence".

Level of quality	Description
• **High**	Very confident that the true effect lies close to that of the estimate of the effect.
• **Moderate**	Moderate confidence in the effect estimate: the true effect is likely to be close to the estimate of the effect, but there is a possibility that it is substantially different.
• **Low**	Limited confidence in the effect estimate: the true effect may be substantially different from the estimate of the effect.
• **Very low**	Little confidence in the effect estimate: the true effect is likely to be substantially different from the estimate of the effect.

4. RESULTS

4.1. Eligible systematic reviews/meta-analyses

Initial search identified 1608 records from electronic databases. Duplicate publications were removed, the remaining 840 records were screened by titles and abstracts to be evaluated for eligibility criteria. At this step, 436 studies that had different topic of interest and 372 studies that had different design were excluded, whereas 32 studies were retrieved in full text for further evaluation of the eligibility.

Finally, 12 articles that did not met the predefined criteria were excluded (Table 9), the remaining 20 articles (72-91) were assessed for quality and used for data synthesis. Figure 1 depicts the study selection process.

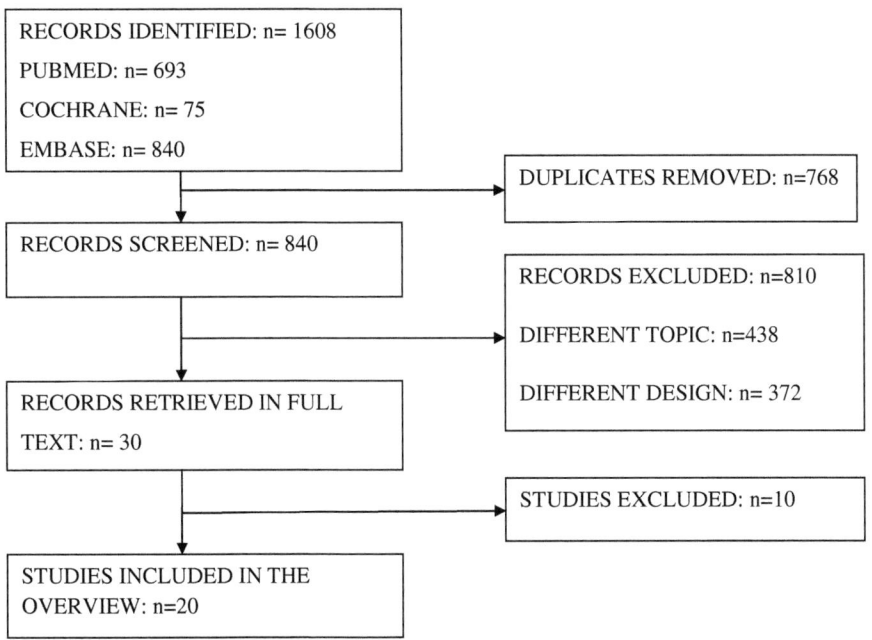

Figure 1. PRISMA flow-chart of study selection.

Table 9. Main reason for exclusion of studies after full text reading.

Article	Reason
Rulli E, Biagioli E, Riva I, Gambirasio G, De Simone I, Floriani I,et al. Efficacy and safety of trabeculectomy vs nonpenetrating surgical procedures: a systematic review and meta-analysis. JAMA Ophthalmol. 2013 Dec;131(12):1573-82.	Included observational studies and ACG patients.
Cheng JW, Cheng SW, Cai JP, Li Y, Wei RL. Systematic overview of the efficacy of nonpenetrating glaucoma surgery in the treatment of open angle glaucoma. Med Sci Monit. 2011 Jul;17(7):RA155-63.	Included also secondary OAG patients.
Qian ZG, Ke M, Huang G, Zou J. Efficacy and safety of latanoprost versus travoprost for primary open-angle glaucoma and ocular hypertension: A meta-analysis. Chin J EBM 2011;11:965-70.	Manuscript entirely in Chinese.
Ting NS, Li Yim JF, Ng JY. Different strategies and cost-effectiveness in the treatment of primary open angle glaucoma. Clinicoecon Outcomes Res. 2014 Dec 4;6:523-30.	A narrative review.
Beidoe G, Mousa SA.Current primary open-angle glaucoma treatments and future directions. Clin Ophthalmol 2012;6:1699-707.	A narrative review.
Librando A, Migliorini R, Pacella F, Turchetti P, Cerutti F, Mazzeo G, et al. Pneumotrabeculoplasty as treatment for primary open angle glaucoma: critical review of the literature. Clin Ter. 2012;163(5):e269-77.	A narrative review.
Ormrod D, McClellan K. Topical dorzolamide 2%/timolol 0.5%: a review of its use in the treatment of open-angle glaucoma. Drugs Aging. 2000 Dec;17(6):477-96.	A narrative review.
Sanfilippo P. A review of argon and selective laser trabeculoplasty as primary treatments of open-angle glaucoma. Clin Exp Optom. 1999 Nov-Dec;82(6):225-229.	A narrative review.
Burr J, Azuara-Blanco A, Avenell A, Tuulonen A. Medical versus surgical interventions for open angle glaucoma. Cochrane Database Syst Rev. 2012 Sep 12;9:CD004399.	Surgical interventions were compared to pilocarpine, now rarely used as first-line medication in POAG.
Sycha T, Vass C, Findl O, Bauer P, Groke I, Schmetterer L, Eichler HG. Interventions for normal tension glaucoma.Cochrane Database Syst Rev. 2010 Feb 17;(2):CD002222.	Withdrawn from publication-outdated.

4.2. Characteristics of systematic reviews/meta-analyses

All included systematic reviews/meta-analyses were published between 2000 and 2014. The objectives, criteria for selection of primary studies and methods used to evaluate and combine data varied.

Twelve of them (74, 75, 78, 79,81-86, 88, 90) evaluated both efficacy and safety, seven evaluated only efficacy (72,73,76, 80, 87, 89, 91), one addressed specifically safety (77), whereas none addressed cost-effectiveness profile of treatments.

Surgical procedures were compared just in one systematic review/meta-analysis (74), while all others evaluated pharmaceutical treatments either as individual (72, 75-84, 86-91) or combined compounds (72, 73, 75, 86). Some treatment modalities, especially laser and surgical procedures, were not included in any of these systematic reviews/meta-analyses. Doses, formulations and dosing regimens of specific drugs differed and were sometimes counted as a single drug.

In general, systematic reviews/meta-analyses included randomized controlled trials (RCTs) and assessed them for quality. Only two of them (75, 87) did not assess the quality of RCTs, while others implemented Cochrane, Delphi or Jadad tools.

More than 85% of patients included across primary studies in systematic reviews were POAG, some did include also individuals with OHT (72, 73, 75-79, 82-89, 91).

In eighteen systematic reviews (72-74, 77-91) data were combined using meta-analysis, whereas in two (75, 76) they were synthesized using network meta-analysis. Four of them were conducted by Cheng et al. (73, 79, 80, 83), and two others by Van der Valk et al. (76, 89).

General characteristics of the 20 included systematic reviews/meta-analyses are provided in Table 10. Since some of them (75-84, 86-91) were already evaluated by an overview in 2014 (57), data regarding their AMSTAR score and GRADE level were extracted from the overview.

Table 10. General characteristics of the included systematic reviews/meta-analyses.

Ref.	Objective	Criteria	Number of studies	Assessments
72	Assess FCLT vs their individual components.	RCT or cross-over; POAG or OHT; Compare FCLT with the mono therapy or UFCLT.	FCLT vs. TIM=8; FCLT vs. LAT=9; FCLT vs. UFCLT=3.	Efficacy: VF defects; optic atrophy; the mean IOP; the fluctuation of IOP.
73	Evaluate fixed-combination drugs that contain TIM.	RCT; POAG/OHT>85%. DORZ/TIM; BRINZ/TIM; BRIM/TIM; LAT/TIM; TRAV/TIM;BIMA/TIM.	DORZ/TIM=22; BRINZ/TIM=2; BRIM/TIM=5; LAT/TIM=14; TRAV/TIM=8; BIMA/TIM=2.	Efficacy: absolute and relative IOP reduction.
74	Compare NPTS and TB.	RCT; OAG not responded to drugs; Compare NPTS with TB.	9	Efficacy: IOP reduction, success rate; Safety: post-op complications.
75	Compare different treatments.	RCT; POAG/OHT; Include a PGA in at least one arm.	73: Placebo; TIM; BIMA; LAT-TIM; CAI-TIM; TRAV-TIM; TRAV; LAT; CAI; Other UC; Other β-blockers.	Efficacy: absolute IOP; predicted probability of IOP <20 mmHg or ≥20% reduction; Safety: patients % with local hyperaemia.
76	Compare the most prescribed mono compounds.	RCT; POAG-HTG or OHT; Compare (any): Placebo; TIM; BET; BRIM; DORZ; BRINZ; LAT; TRAV; BIMA .	BIMA=6; BET=5; LAT=12;TRAV=5; TIM=15;BRIM=4; BRINZ=1; DORZ=6.	Efficacy: absolute and relative IOP reduction for peak and trough using TIM as a reference.
77	Compare LAT with BIMA and TRAV.	RCT; Glaucoma/OHT; Any comparison between LAT, BIMA or TRAV.	LAT vs. BIMA=8; LAT vs. TRAV=6; 3 arms=1.	Safety: Conjunctival hyperaemia.
78	Compare BIMA, LAT and TRAV.	RCT; POAG/OHT; Any comparison between TRAV, LAT and BIMA.	TRAV vs. LAT=9; LAT vs. BIMA=8; TRAV vs BIMA=8.	Efficacy: IOP at study end; Safety: hyperaemia of conjunctiva.
79	Compare TRAV and LAT .	RCT; OAG/OHT with IOP >21 mmHg; Compare TRAV to LAT.	17	Efficacy: IOP reduction; Safety: local and AE withdrawals.

Ref.	Objective	Criteria	Number of studies	Assessments
80	Compare the most prescribed mono compounds.	RCT; Advanced NPG; Compare (any): Placebo; BET; TIM; DORZ; BRINZ; BRIM; LAT; TRAV; BIMA.	15	Efficacy: absolute and relative IOP reduction for peak, trough and diurnal curve for each drug.
81	Compare TIM with BRIM.	RCT, Glaucoma; Directly compare TIM to BRIM.	10	Efficacy: IOP reduction; Safety: local, systemic.
82	Compare PGA with BRIM and DORZ.	RCT; OAG/OHT, ACG excluded; Compare PGAs and BRIM or DORZ.	LAT vs BRIM=4; LAT vs DORZ=3.	Efficacy: IOP reduction; Safety: local, AE withdrawals.
83	Compare BIMA with LAT.	RCT; Glaucoma or OHT, Directly compare LAT and BIMA.	13	Efficacy: IOP reduction or % of patients achieving IOP≤17; Safety. Local.
84	Compare BIMA, LAT and TRAV.	RCT; POAG /OHT >90%; Compare LAT, TRAV or BIMA.	LAT vs BIMA=4; LAT vs TRAV=1; TRAV vs BIMA=2	Efficacy: IOP reduction; Safety: conjunctival hyperaemia.
85	Compare the topical medications.	RCT; POAG or OHT Compare any topical pharmacological treatment to placebo, no treatment or other treatment.	26; Meta-analysis=10 .	Efficacy: reduction of onset or progression of VF or RNFL loss, ONH cupping progression; and improvement of VF; Safety: local and systemic.
86	Compare LAT with BRIM .	RCT; OAG/NTG/OHT; Compare LAT to BRIM; adjunctive treatment possible.	15 Mono-treatment=9; Adjunctive=6.	Efficacy: peak or diurnal IOP reduction; Safety: local and systemic.
87	Compare TRAV with LAT and BIMA.	RCT; OAG or OHT; Any comparison of TRAV, LAT, BIMA.	9; Comparing all 3=2; Comparing two =7.	Efficacy: IOP reduction and % responding for each individual treatment.
88	Compare TRAV with LAT, BIMA and TIM.	RCT; OAG or OHT; Compare TRAV vs. other PGA or TIM.	TRAV vs. TIM=4; TRAV vs. LAT=5; TRAV vs BIMA=5.	Efficacy: ΔIOP vs. baseline; Safety: local.

Ref.	Objective	Criteria	Number of studies	Assessments
89	Compare the most prescribed mono compounds.	RCT; POAG-HTG or OHT; Compare (any): Placebo; TIM; BET; BRIM; DORZ; BRINZ; LAT; TRAV; BIMA.	Placebo=3; BET=5; BRIM=4; TIM=15;BIMA=6; LAT=12; DORZ=6; TRAV=5; BRINZ=1.	Efficacy: absolute and relative ΔIOP vs. baseline for peak and trough for each individual treatment.
90	Indirectly compare LAT with BRIM.	RCT; POAG with IOP $\geq$20 mmHg; At least one arm includes LAT or BRIM.	LAT=6; BRIM=3.	Efficacy: IOP reduction and % with controlled IOP for LAT and BRIM.
91	Compare LAT with TIM.	RCT; OAG/OHT; Directly compare LAT and TIM.	11	Efficacy: IOP reduction; Safety: local, systemic, AE withdrawals.

* Data regarding some systematic reviews/meta-analyses are extracted from the overview published in 2014 (57).

RCT = Randomized Controlled Trial; POAG = Primary Open Angle Glaucoma;

OHT = Ocular Hypertension; NTG = Normal Tension Glaucoma; OAG = Open Angle Glaucoma;

ACG = Angle Closed Glaucoma; HTG = High Tension Glaucoma; IOP = Intraocular Pressure;

AEs = Adverse Events; VF= Visual Field; RNFL= Retinal Nerve Fibre Layer; ONH = Optic Nerve Head;

PGAs = Prostaglandin Analogues; CAI = Carbonic Anhydrase Inhibitors; TRAV = Travoprost;

UC = Unfixed Combinations; LAT = Latanoprost; BIMA = Bimatoprost; BRIM = Brimonidine;

TIM = Timolol; BET = Betaxolol; DORZ = Dorzolamide; BRINZ = Brinzolamide; TB= Trabeculectomy,

FCLT = Fixed Combination of Latanoprost and Timolol; NPTS = Non-Penetrating Trabecular Surgery;

UFCLT= Unfixed Combination of Latanoprost and Timolol.

4.3. Methodological quality of systematic reviews/meta-analyses

Methodological quality of the included systematic reviews/meta-analyses, evaluated by the AMSTAR checklist, is summarized in Table 11. Only two of them (72, 85) achieved an overall methodological quality level of 11 points, while the others scored between 7 and 10 points.

One systematic review/meta-analysis (87) was downgraded for the second AMSTAR item as the process of study selection and data abstraction was not conducted by two reviewers, in two others (74, 75) there was a lack of information to decide about this item.

Only four systematic reviews/meta-analyses (72, 75, 77, 83, 85, 88) provided the list of both included and excluded studies, whereas others provided only the list of the included studies and were not checked for the fifth AMSTAR item.

Quality of the included primary studies was not assessed in two systematic reviews/meta-analyses (75, 87), therefore they were downgraded for the seventh AMSTAR item.

Six systematic reviews/meta-analyses (75-77, 83, 88, 89) were downgraded for the eighth AMSTAR item because the quality of primary studies was not accounted for conclusions.

Appropriate pooling methods were applied only in six systematic reviews/meta-analyses (72, 75, 78, 82, 85, 86), whereas others used fixed-effects pooling instead of random-effects; pooled values for individual treatments across trials or used erroneous method to calculate SD of change in IOP vs. baseline, therefore were downgraded for the ninth AMSTAR item.

Tenth AMSTAR item was not fulfilled by five systematic reviews/meta-analyses (82, 83, 89-91) as publication bias was not assessed, whereas the eleventh item was not fulfilled by four systematic reviews/meta-analyses(74, 79, 81, 90) because authors did not declare the conflict of interest.

Table 11. AMSTAR methodological quality score of systematic reviews/meta-analyses.

Ref.	72	73	74	75	76	77	78	79	80	81	82	83	84	85	86	87	88	89	90	91
D	Y	Y	Y	Y	Y	Y	Y	Y	10	Y	Y	Y	Y	Y	Y	Y	Y	Y	Y	Y
S/E	Y	Y	?	?	Y	Y	Y	Y	Y	Y	Y	Y	Y	Y	Y	N	Y	Y	Y	Y
S	Y	Y	Y	Y	Y	Y	Y	Y	Y	Y	Y	Y	Y	Y	Y	Y	Y	Y	Y	Y
P	Y	Y	Y	Y	Y	Y	Y	Y	Y	Y	Y	Y	Y	Y	Y	Y	Y	Y	Y	Y
L	Y	?	?	Y	?	Y	?	?	?	?	?	Y	?	Y	?	?	Y	?	?	?
CH	Y	Y	Y	Y	Y	Y	Y	Y	Y	Y	Y	Y	Y	Y	Y	Y	Y	Y	Y	Y
Q	Y	Y	Y	N	Y	Y	Y	Y	Y	Y	Y	Y	Y	Y	Y	N	Y	Y	Y	Y
C	Y	Y	Y	N	N	N	Y	Y	Y	Y	Y	N	Y	Y	Y	N	N	Y	Y	Y
M	Y	?	?	Y	?	?	Y	N	N	N	Y	?	?	Y	Y	N	?	N	N	N
B	Y	Y	Y	Y	Y	Y	Y	Y	Y	Y	N	N	Y	Y	Y	Y	Y	N	N	N
I	Y	Y	N	Y	Y	Y	Y	N	Y	N	Y	Y	Y	Y	Y	Y	Y	Y	N	Y
Score	11	9	7	8	8	9	10	8	9	8	9	8	9	11	10	6	9	8	7	8

* Data regarding some systematic reviews/meta-analyses are extracted from the overview published in 2014 (57).

D = Study design; S/E = Duplicate Selection/Extraction; S= Comprehensive Search;
P = Publication Status; L = List of studies; CH = Characteristics of studies; Q = Quality of studies;
C =Conclusions; M = Methods of pooling; B = Publication Bias; I = Conflict of interest.

4.4. Evidence quality

Table 12 depicts the quality of the evidence provided by the included systematic reviews/meta-analyses (where each one is a "body of evidence") as assigned by GRADE framework. Assessment of the GRADE quality level was based on the properties of the primary trials included, as well as precision of the estimates and type of treatment comparisons within systematic reviews/meta-analyses.

Since none of the included systematic reviews/meta-analyses provided evidence of high quality, evaluation of IOP lowering modalities for POAG treatment was based on seven of them (72, 75, 77, 84-86, 88) that provided evidence of moderate quality as assessed by the GRADE evaluation system.

Some systematic reviews/meta-analyses, although methodologically well conducted, provided only low or very low quality of evidence. Since the true effect in these studies is likely to be substantially different from the estimate of effects, they were not considered as a confident evidence for evaluation of treatments.

Table 12. Evidence quality level, evaluated by GRADE system.

Ref.	Limitations/ bias	Inconsistency	Indirectness	Imprecision	Publication bias	Quality of evidence
72	-1	Some	Direct	Some	Unlikely	**Moderate**
73	-1	-1	-2	Some	Unlikely	**Very Low**
74	-1	Minor	Direct	-1	Unlikely	**Low**
75	Possible	No	-1	Minor	Unlikely	**Moderate**
76	-1	Minor	-1	Minor	Unlikely	**Low**
77	-1	No	Direct	Minor	Unlikely	**Moderate**
78	-2	Some	Direct	Minor	Unlikely	**Low**
79	-1	Minor	Direct	-1	Unlikely	**Low**
80	-1	Minor	-2	Some	Unlikely	**Very Low**
81	-1	-1	Direct	Minor	Unlikely	**Low**
82	-1	Some	Direct	-1	Unlikely	**Low**
83	-1	-1	Direct	Some	Unlikely	**Low**
84	Minor	Minor	Direct	-1	Unlikely	**Moderate**
85	-1	Some	Direct	Some	Unlikely	**Moderate**
86	-1	Minor	Direct	Minor	Unlikely	**Moderate**
87	-2	-1	-2	Minor	Unlikely	**Very Low**
88	Minor	Minor	Direct	-1	Unlikely	**Moderate**
89	-1	Minor	-2	Minor	Unlikely	**Very Low**
90	-1	-1	Direct	Minor	Unlikely	**Low**
91	-1	Minor	-2	Minor	Unlikely	**Very Low**

* Data regarding some systematic reviews/meta-analyses are extracted from the overview published in 2014 (57).

4.5. Evidence on efficacy of IOP-lowering treatments for POAG

All systematic reviews/meta-analyses of moderate quality (72, 75, 77, 84-86, 88) addressed IOP lowering drugs, none provided evidence on laser or surgical IOP lowering procedures. Beside two of them (72, 85) that assessed the effect of drugs on VF, RNFL or ONH, in others, the only assessed outcome for effect was the level of IOP reduction. The evaluated drugs were: β-blockers (timolol, betaxolol, carteolol, levobunolol); CAIs (brinzolamide, dorzolamide), PGAs (latanoprost, travoprost, and bimatoprost) and brimonidine. Some drugs were also evaluated, in combinations, for their effect on POAG patients that were uncontrolled with mono-therapy.

A recent overview (57) that evaluated mono-compound IOP lowering medications, and included some of these systematic reviews/meta-analyses (75, 77, 84, 86, 88), summarized that the IOP reduction difference between mono-compound IOP lowering drugs in OHT/POAG treatment was very small and although statistically significant did not seem practically relevant. In general, PGAs were more effective compared to other drugs, whereas the three PGAs appeared to be equivalent as the IOP reducing potential was in between the limits (-1.0 to +1.0 mmHg) of the therapeutic equivalence (57). However, in regard to IOP lowering effect, evidence from the only systematic review (72) that compared fixed combination of latanoprost and timolol (FCLT) to their individual components or unfixed combination (UCLT) showed that the effect of combined therapy was significantly higher compared to individual treatments.

Evidence regarding the effect of IOP lowering drugs in VF and ONH (72, 85) was insufficient, data for the most of the newer drugs were absent. Overall, the following drugs were addressed: timolol, betaxolol, carteolol, levobunolol, dorzolamide, brimonidine, pilocarpine, epinephrine, latanoprost, and FCLT. Vass et al. (85) could demonstrate that β-blockers had a protective effect on VF, however, the evidence was weak. Furthermore, they could not demonstrate a clear evidence of a beneficial effect for any drug individually. Although Xing at al. (72) aimed to compare FCLT with their individual compounds regarding the VF defects and ONH atrophy, they could not find sufficient evidence to confirm the difference. Limitations in both systematic reviews (72, 85) were raised due to the low quality of the primary studies.

4.6. Evidence on safety of IOP-lowering treatments for POAG

The main assessed outcome for safety of IOP lowering drugs in five systematic reviews/meta-analyses of moderate quality (75, 77, 84, 86, 88) was conjunctival hyperemia, whereas the most common drugs evaluated were PGAs.

All three, evaluated PGAs, had worse profile of hyperaemia compared to timolol, while bimatoprost was considerably worse than timolol, brinzolamide and brimonidine (57). In regard to PGAs, odds of hyperemia with latanoprost were lower compared to travoprost or bimatoprost, whereas evidence on travoprost vs. bimatoprost was inconclusive (57). Difference between the evaluated non-PGAs drugs: brinzolamide, timolol and brimonidine in respect to conjunctival hyperemia was not relevant (75).

Although two systematic reviews (86, 88) provided more evidence on adverse events for: latanoprost, travoporst, brimonidine and timolol, their quality level was lower (57).

The only available evidence on withdrawals due to adverse events was provided by Vass et al.(85). It addressed mainly β-blockers and demonstrated that, within the group, the frequency of withdrawals was significantly larger for timolol compared to betaxolol. In contrary, when compared to brimonidine, timolol had a significantly lower risk of adverse events necessitating cessation of treatment (85).

5. DISCUSSION

Since POAG is the leading cause of irreversible blindness worldwide, its treatment has been extensively investigated. However, still, POAG treatment reveals many questions in regard to the type, regime, benefit, safety and cost-effectiveness profile of treatment modalities.

The present overview addressed only one component of POAG treatment, but the one that is approved by all guidelines - IOP lowering treatment. Within this broad field of evidence, the aim was to evaluate the evidence on the relative efficacy, safety and cost-effectiveness profile of IOP-lowering treatments. This assessment is of practical relevance as:

a) identification of IOP lowering treatments with the best trade-off between efficacy and safety would help optimize the treatment; additionally, identification of modalities with the best cost-effectiveness profile would be particularly useful for developing countries with restricted public health resources;

b) although the current focus of research for POAG treatment is on non-IOP lowering modalities, the identification of new therapeutic targets has been hampered by lack of understanding the POAG aetiology.

5.1. Overall completeness and applicability of evidence

The overview identified a number of systematic reviews/meta-analyses dealing with IOP lowering treatments, but most of them provided a very low level of evidence quality and were not further evaluated. Therefore, data about laser and surgical interventions are missing.

Some older drug classes and newer IOP lowering compounds are not evaluated because they have not been addressed in any systematic review. However, lack of information for these drugs is not of importance as the addressed drugs on this overview have become standards.

Major limitations on the overview arise from the missing of data on cost-effectiveness profile of treatments.

5.2. Quality of evidence

The aims of the overview were very comprehensive, assessing a number of important outcomes related to efficacy and safety of IOP lowering treatments. None of the included systematic reviews/meta-analyses provided evidence of high quality, however, different levels of quality of evidence were established considering efficacy and safety of treatments:

Efficacy: Evidence on relationships in between the three PGAs; between PGAs and non-PGAs; and between FCLT and their individual components or UFCLT in respect to IOP reduction difference was of moderate quality. Evidence on relationships between β-blockers, dorzolamide, brimonidine, pilocarpine, epinephrine, latanoprost, and FCLT in respect to VF or ONH changes was of low quality and inconclusive;

Safety: Evidence on relationships in between the three PGAs; between PGAs, timolol, brinzolamide and brimonidine in respect to conjunctival hyperaemia was of moderate quality. Evidence on relationships in between β-blockers or between latanoprost, travoporst, brimonidine and timolol in respect to other adverse events or withdrawals due to adverse events was of less than moderate quality.

5.3. Potential biases in the overview process

Protection from bias in this overview was achieved by a thorough literature search and evidence assessment. When the overall body of evidence was not at least of moderate quality any conclusions were avoided. In this way, were avoided potential biases that could have been introduced by low-quality primary studies or systematic reviews/meta-analysis.

However, during the overview process, individual primary studies for treatment modalities that have not been a part of any systematic review were not included. Omission of those data could have raised major biases on the overview.

6. CONCLUSIONS

Despite a number of individual studies and systematic reviews available and continuous research interest in the field of POAG treatment, many questions still remain unanswered. In general, available evidence for most of the IOP lowering treatment modalities does not derive from high quality systematic reviews, therefore data do not provide the basis for sound conclusions. Furthermore yet, high quality primary studies for laser and surgical interventions but also for newer IOP lowering drugs have not been a subject of systematic reviews/meta-analyses.

6.1. Implications for practice

Although treatments were not ranked based on efficacy, safety or cost-effective profile in any systematic review, data from a recent overview (57) suggest that PGAs emerge as preferred mono-compound treatments for POAG and among them latanoprost has the most favourable trade-off between efficacy and tolerability.

In case when PGAs are contraindicated, there is no clear evidence that supports the superiority of any non-PGA compound either in regard to efficacy or safety. Whereas, in respect to elevated IOP, both fixed and unfixed combinations of latanoprost and timolol had higher effect compared to their individual compounds on POAG patients that were uncontrolled with mono-therapy.

6.2. Implications for research

A large number of IOP lowering treatments have been addressed in systematic reviews over the years, but most of them apparently only superficially. However, for most of the current standard drugs, there is actually an amount of high quality primary trials that could be converted into evidence of relevant quality with appropriate implementation of data-pooling techniques.

High quality RTCs should be designed to assess the efficacy and safety of laser and surgical interventions.

7. REFERENCES

1.Cherecheanu AP, Garhofer G, Schmidl D, Werkmeister R, Schmetterer L. Ocular perfusion pressure and ocular blood flow in glaucoma. Curr Opin Pharmacol. 2013;13:36-42.

2. Kanski JJ, Bowling B. Clinical Ophthalmology: a systematic approach. 7th edition. Elsevier, 2011.

3. Pascolini D, Mariotti SP. Global estimates of visual impairment: 2010. Br J Ophthalmol. 2012;96:614-8.

4. Mowatt G, Burr JM, Cook JA, Siddiqui MA, Ramsay C, Fraser C, et al. Screening tests for detecting open-angle glaucoma: systematic review and meta-analysis. Invest Ophthalmol Vis Sci. 2008;49:5373-85.

5. Quigley HA, Broman AT. The number of people with glaucoma worldwide in 2010 and 2020. Br J Ophthalmol. 2006;90:262–7.

6. Resnikoff S, Pascolini D, Etya'ale D, Kocur I, Pararajasegaram R, Pokharel, et al. Global data on visual impairment in the year 2002. Bull World Health Organ. 2004;82:844–51.

7. Burr JM, Mowatt G, Hernandez R, et al. The clinical effectiveness and cost-effectiveness of screening for open angle glaucoma: a systematic review and economic evaluation. Health Technol Assess. 2007;11:1–190.

8. Rudnicka AR, Mt-Isa S, Owen CG, Cook DG, Ashby D. Variations in Primary Open-Angle Glaucoma Prevalence by Age, Gender, and Race: A Bayesian Meta-Analysis. Invest Ophthalmol Vis Sci. 2006;47:4254-61.

9. Kroese M, Burton H. Primary open angle glaucoma. The need for a consensus case definition. J Epidemiol Community Health. 2003;57:752-4.

10. American Academy of Ophthalmology Preferred Practice Patterns Committee. Preferred Practice Pattern® Guidelines. Primary Open-Angle Glaucoma. San Francisco, CA: American Academy of Ophthalmology; 2010.

11. European Glaucoma Society. Terminology and guidelines for glaucoma, 3rd Edition. Savona, Italy: Dogma, 2008.

12. Shields M. Normal-tension glaucoma: is it different from primary open-angle glaucoma? Curr Opin Ophthalmol. 2008;19:85-88.

13. Thonginnetra O, Greenstein VC, Chu D, Liebmann JM, Ritch R, Hood DC. Normal versus high tension glaucoma: a comparison of functional and structural defects. J Glaucoma. 2010;19:151-57.

14. Asrani S, Samuels B, Thakur M, Santiago C, Kuchibhatla M. Clinical Profiles of Primary Open Angle Glaucoma versus Normal Tension Glaucoma Patients: A Pilot Study. Curr Eye Res. 2011;36:429-35.

15. Shields MB, Spaeth GL. The Glaucomatous Process and the Evolving Definition of Glaucoma. J Glaucoma 2011;21:141-3.

16. Lichter PR, Musch DC, Gillespie BW, Guire KE, Janz NK, Wren PA, Mills RP; CIGTS Study Group. Interim clinical outcomes in the Collaborative Initial Glaucoma Treatment Study comparing initial treatment randomized to medications or surgery. Ophthalmology. 2001;108:1943-53.

17. Johnson DH. Progress in glaucoma: early detection new treatments, less blindness. Ophthalmology. 2003;110:634-5.

18. American Academy of Ophthalmology Preferred Practice Patterns Committee. Preferred Practice Pattern® Guidelines. Primary Open-Angle Glaucoma Suspect. San Francisco, CA: American Academy of Ophthalmology; 2010.

19. Cioffi, G. A. 2011-2012 Basic and Clinical Science Course, Section 10. Glaucoma.1 edition. American Academy of Ophthalmology, 2011.

20. Bathija R, Gupta N, Zangwill L, Weinreb RN. Changing definition of glaucoma. J Glaucoma. 1998;7:165-9.

21. Sommer A. Ocular Hypertension and Normal-Tension Glaucoma: Time for Banishment and Burial. Arch Ophthalmol. 2011;129:785-7.

22. Giaconi JA, Law SK, Coleman AL, Caprioli, J. Pearls of Glaucoma Management. Springer-Verlag, 2010

23. Schacknow PN, Samples JR. The Glaucoma Book: A Practical, Evidence-Based Approach to Patient Care. Springer, 2010.

24. Mozaffarieh M, Flammer J. Ocular Blood Flow and Glaucomatous Optic Neuropathy. Springer, 2009.

25. Bhan A, Browning AC, Shah S, Hamilton R, Dave D, Dua HS. Effect of corneal thickness on intraocular pressure measurements with the pneumotonometer, Goldmann applanation tonometer, and Tono-Pen. Invest Ophthalmol Vis Sci. 2002;43:1389-92.

26. Jonas JB, Gusek GC, Naumann GO. Optic disc morphometry in chronic primary open-angle glaucoma. Graefes Arch Clin Exp Ophthalmol. 1988;226:522-30.

27. Jonas JB, Fernández MC, Stürmer J. Patterns of glaucomatous neuroretinal rim loss. Ophthalmology. 1993;100:63-8.

28. Azuara-Blanco A, Costa VP, Wilson RP. Handbook of glaucoma. Martin Dunitz, 2003.

29. Osborne NN, Melena J, Chidlow G, Wood JPM. A hypothesis to explain ganglion cell death caused by vascular insults at the optic nerve head: possible implication for the treatment of glaucoma. Br JOphthalmol. 2001;85:1252-9.

30. Flammer J, Mozaffarieh M. What Is the Present Pathogenetic Concept of Glaucomatous Optic Neuropathy? Surv Ophthalmol. 2007;52:S162-73.

31. American Academy of Ophthalmology Preferred Practice Patterns Committee. Preferred Practice Pattern® Guidelines. Comprehensive Adult Medical Eye Evaluation. San Francisco, CA: American Academy of Ophthalmology; 2010.

32. Crabb DP, Smith ND, Glen FC, Burton R, Garway-Heath DF. How does glaucoma look?: patient perception of visual field loss. Ophthalmology. 2013;120:1120-6.

33. Barkana Y, Anis S, Liebmann J, Tello C, Ritch R. Clinical utility of intraocular pressure monitoring outside of normal office hours in patients with glaucoma. Arch Ophthalmol. 2006;124:793-7.

34. Hasegawa K, Ishida K, Sawada A, Kawase K, Yamamoto T. Diurnal variation of intraocular pressure in suspected normal-tension glaucoma. Jpn J Ophthalmol. 2006;50:449-54.

35. Bagga H, Liu JH, Weinreb RN. Intraocular pressure measurements throughout the 24 h. Curr Opin Ophthalmol 2009;20:79-83.

36. Brandt JD. The influence of corneal thickness on the diagnosis and management of glaucoma. J Glaucoma. 2001;10;S6-7.

37. Liu J, Roberts CJ. Influence of corneal biomechanical properties on intraocular pressure measurement quantitative analysis. J Cataract Refract Surg. 2005;31:146–55.

38. Touboul D, Roberts C, Kerautret J, Garra C, Maurice-Tison S, Saubusse E, et al. Correlations between corneal hysteresis, intraocular pressure, and corneal central pachymetry. J Cataract Refract Surg. 2008;34:616–22.

39. Alward WLM. Color Atlas of Gonioscopy. San Francisco: Foundation of the American Academy of Ophthalmology; 2000.

40. Iester M, Zingirian M. Quality of life in patients with early, moderate and advanced glaucoma. Eye (Lond). 2002;16:44-9.

41. Nelson P, Aspinall P, Papasouliotis O, Worton B, O'Brien C. Quality of life in glaucoma and its relationship with visual function. J Glaucoma. 2003;12:139-50.

42. Spry PG, Johnson CA. Identification of progressive glaucomatous visual field loss. Surv Ophthalmol. 2002;47:158-73.

43. Graham SL, Klistorner AL. Goldberg I. Clinical application of objective perimetry using multifocal visual evoked potentials in glaucoma practice. Arch Ophthalmol. 2005;123:729-39.

44. Schmetterer L, Garhofer G. How can blood flow be measured? Surv Ophthalmol. 2007;52:S134–8.

45. Kass MA, Heuer DK, Higginbotham EJ, Johnson CA, Keltner JL, Miller JP, et al. The Ocular Hypertension Treatment Study: a randomized trial determines that topical ocular hypotensive medication delays or prevents the onset of primary open-angle glaucoma. Arch Ophthalmol. 2002;120:701-13.

46. Heijl A, Leske MC, Bengtsson B, Hyman L, Bengtsson B, Hussein M; Early Manifest Glaucoma Trial Group. Reduction of intraocular pressure and glaucoma progression: results from the Early Manifest Glaucoma Trial. Arch Ophthalmol. 2002;120:1268-79.

47. Osborne NN, del Olmo-Aguado S. Maintenance of retinal ganglion cell mitochondrial functions as a neuroprotective strategy in glaucoma. Curr Opin Pharmacol. 2013;13:16-22.

48. Beidoe G, Mousa SA. Current primary open-angle glaucoma treatments and future directions. Clin Ophthalmol. 2012;6:1699-707.

49. Lee DA, Higginbotham EJ. Glaucoma and its treatment: a review. Am J Health Syst Pharm. 2005;62:691-9.

50. Whitson JT. Glaucoma: a review of adjunctive therapy and new management strategies. Expert Opin Pharmacother. 2007;8:3237-49.

51. Marquis RE, Whitson JT. Management of glaucoma: focus on pharmacological therapy. Drugs Aging. 2005;22:1-21.

52. Netland PA; Ophthalmic Technology Assessment Committee Glaucoma Panel, American Academy of Ophthalmology. Nonpenetrating glaucoma surgery. Ophthalmology. 2001;108:416-21.

53. Honjo M, Tanihara T, Inatani M, Honda Y, Ogino N, Ueno S, et al. Phacoemulsification, intraocular lens implantation, and trabeculotomy to treat pseudoexfoliation syndrome. J Cataract Refract Surg. 1998;24:781-6.

54. Hattenhauer MG, Johnson DH, Ing HH, Herman DC, Hodge DO, Yawn BP, et al. The probability of blindness from open-angle glaucoma. Ophthalmology. 1998;105:2099-104.

55. Grehn F, Stamper R. Glaucoma Essentials in Ophthalmology. Springer. 2009.

56. Maynard A. Ethics and health care 'underfunding'. Med Ethics. 2001;27:223-7.

57. Daka Q, Trkulja V. Efficacy and tolerability of mono-compound topical treatments for reduction of intraocular pressure in patients with primary open angle glaucoma or ocular hypertension: an overview of reviews. Croat Med J. 2014 Oct;55(5):468-80.

58. Higgins JPT, Green S (editors). Cochrane Handbook for Systematic Reviews of Interventions, version 5.1.0 [updated March 2011]. The Cochrane Collaboration, 2011. Available from www.cochrane-handbook.org. Accessed: November 20, 2011.

59. Moher D, Liberati A, Tetzlaff J, Altman DG, The PRISMA Group (2009). Preferred Reporting Items for Systematic Reviews and Meta-Analyses: The PRISMA Statement. BMJ 2009;339:b2535.

60. Shea BJ, Hamel C, Wells GA, Bouter LM, Kristjansson E, Grimshaw J, et al. AMSTAR is a reliable and valid measurement tool to assess the methodological quality of systematic reviews. J Clin Epidemiol. 2009;62:1013-20.

61. Shea BJ, Grimshaw JM, Wells GA, Boers M, Andersson N, Hamel C, et al. Development of AMSTAR: a measurement tool to assess the methodological quality of systematic reviews. BMC Med Res Methodol. 2007;7:10.

62. Guyatt GH, Oxman AD, Kunz R, Vist GE, Falck-Ytter Y, Schünemann HJ; GRADE Working Group. What is "quality of evidence" and why is it important to clinicians? BMJ. 2008;336:995-8.

63. Guyatt G, Oxman AD, Akl EA, Kunz R, Vist G, Brozek J, et al. GRADE guidelines: 1. Introduction-GRADE evidence profiles and summary of findings tables. J Clin Epidemiol. 2011;64:383-94.

64. Guyatt GH, Oxman AD, Kunz R, Atkins D, Brozek J, Vist G, et al. GRADE guidelines: 2. Framing the question and deciding on important outcomes. J Clin Epidemiol. 2011;64:395-400.

65. Balshem H, Helfand M, Schünemann HJ, Oxman AD, Kunz R, Brozek J, et al. GRADE guidelines: 3. Rating the quality of evidence. J Clin Epidemiol. 2011;64:401-6.

66. Guyatt GH, Oxman AD, Vist G, Kunz R, Brozek J, Alonso-Coello P, et al. GRADE guidelines: 4. Rating the quality of evidence-study limitations (risk of bias). J Clin Epidemiol. 2011;64:407-15.

67. Guyatt GH, Oxman AD, Montori V, Vist G, Kunz R, Brozek J, et al. GRADE guidelines: 5. Rating the quality of evidence-publication bias. J Clin Epidemiol. 2011;64:1277-82.

68. Guyatt GH, Oxman AD, Kunz R, Brozek J, Alonso-Coello P, Rind D, et al. GRADE guidelines 6. Rating the quality of evidence-imprecision. J Clin Epidemiol. 2011;64:1283-93.

69. Guyatt GH, Oxman AD, Kunz R, Woodcock J, Brozek J, Helfand M, et al. GRADE guidelines: 7. Rating the quality of evidence-inconsistency. J Clin Epidemiol. 2011;64:1294-302.

70. Guyatt GH, Oxman AD, Kunz R, Woodcock J, Brozek J, Helfand M, et al. GRADE guidelines: 8. Rating the quality of evidence-indirectness. J Clin Epidemiol. 2011;64:1303-10.

71. Guyatt GH, Oxman AD, Sultan S, Glasziou P, Akl EA, Alonso-Coello P, et al. GRADE guidelines: 9. Rating up the quality of evidence. J Clin Epidemiol. 2011;64:1311-6.

72. Xing Y, Jiang FG, Li T. Fixed combination of latanoprost and timolol vs the individual components for primary open angle glaucoma and ocular hypertension: a systematic review and meta-analysis. Int J Ophthalmol. 2014 Oct 18;7(5):879-90.

73.Cheng JW, Cheng SW, Gao LD, Lu GC, Wei RL. Intraocular pressure-lowering effects of commonly used fixed-combination drugs with timolol: a systematic review and meta-analysis. PLoS One. 2012;7(9):e45079.

74. Ke M, Guo J, Qian Z. Meta analysis of non-penetrating trabecular surgery versus trabeculectomy for the treatment of open angle glaucoma. J Huazhong Univ Sci Technolog Med Sci. 2011 Apr;31(2):264-70.

75. Orme M, Collins S, Dakin H, Kelly S, Loftus J. Mixed treatment comparison and meta-regression of the efficacy and safety of prostaglandin analogues and comparators for primary open-angle glaucoma and ocular hypertension. Curr Med Res Opin. 2010;26:511-28.

76. van der Valk R, Webers CA, Lumley T, Hendrikse F, Prins MH, Schouten JS. A network meta-analysis combined direct and indirect comparisons between glaucoma drugs to rank effectiveness in lowering intraocular pressure. J Clin Epidemiol. 2009;62:1279-83.

77. Honrubia F, García-Sánchez J, Polo V, de la Casa JM, Soto J. Conjunctival hyperaemia with the use of latanoprost versus other prostaglandin analogues in patients with ocular hypertension or glaucoma: a meta-analysis of randomised clinical trials. Br J Ophthalmol. 2009;93:316-21.

78. Eyawo O, Nachega J, Lefebvre P, Meyer D, Rachlis B, Lee CW, et al. Efficacy and safety of prostaglandin analogues in patients with predominantly primary open-angle glaucoma or ocular hypertension: a meta-analysis. Clin Ophthalmol. 2009;3:447-56.

79. Cheng JW, Xi GL, Wei RL, Cai JP, Li Y. Effects of travoprost in the treatment of open-angle glaucoma or ocular hypertension: A systematic review and meta-analysis. Curr Ther Res Clin Exp. 2009;70:335-50.

80. Cheng JW, Cai JP, Wei RL. Meta-analysis of medical intervention for normal tension glaucoma. Ophthalmology. 2009;116:1243-9.

81. Loon SC, Liew G, Fung A, Reid SE, Craig JC. Meta-analysis of randomized controlled trials comparing timolol with brimonidine in the treatment of glaucoma. Clin Experiment Ophthalmol. 2008;36:281-9.

82. Hodge WG, Lachaine J, Steffensen I, Murray C, Barnes D, Foerster V, et al. The efficacy and harm of prostaglandin analogues for IOP reduction in glaucoma patients compared to dorzolamide and brimonidine: a systematic review. Br J Ophthalmol. 2008;92:7-12.

83. Cheng JW, Wei RL. Meta-analysis of 13 randomized controlled trials comparing bimatoprost with latanoprost in patients with elevated intraocular pressure. Clin Ther. 2008;30:622-32.

84. Aptel F, Cucherat M, Denis P. Efficacy and tolerability of prostaglandin analogs: a meta-analysis of randomized controlled clinical trials. J Glaucoma. 2008;17:667-73.

85. Vass C, Hirn C, Sycha T, Findl O, Bauer P, Schmetterer L. Medical interventions for primary open angle glaucoma and ocular hypertension. Cochrane Database Syst Rev. 2007 Oct 17;(4):CD003167.

86. Fung AT, Reid SE, Jones MP, Healey PR, McCluskey PJ, Craig JC. Meta-analysis of randomised controlled trials comparing latanoprost with brimonidine in the treatment of open-angle glaucoma, ocular hypertension or normal-tension glaucoma. Br J Ophthalmol. 2007;91:62-8.

87. Denis P, Lafuma A, Khoshnood B, Mimaud V, Berdeaux G. A meta-analysis of topical prostaglandin analogues intra-ocular pressure lowering in glaucoma therapy. Curr Med Res Opin. 2007;23:601-8.

88. Li N, Chen XM, Zhou Y, Wei ML, Yao X. Travoprost compared with other prostaglandin analogues or timolol in patients with open-angle glaucoma or ocular hypertension: meta-analysis of randomized controlled trials. Clin Experiment Ophthalmol. 2006;34:755-64.

89. van der Valk R, Webers CA, Schouten JS, Zeegers MP, Hendrikse F, Prins MH. Intraocular pressure-lowering effects of all commonly used glaucoma drugs: a meta-analysis of randomized clinical trials. Ophthalmology. 2005;112:1177-85.

90. Zhang WY, Po AL, Dua HS, Azuara-Blanco A. Meta-analysis of randomised controlled trials comparing latanoprost with timolol in the treatment of patients with open angle glaucoma or ocular hypertension. Br J Ophthalmol. 2001;85:983-90.

91. Einarson TR, Kulin NA, Tingey D, Iskedjian M. Meta-analysis of the effect of latanoprost and brimonidine on intraocular pressure in the treatment of glaucoma. Clin Ther. 2000;22:1502-15.

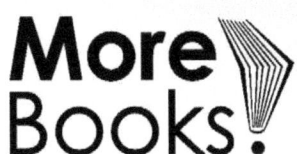
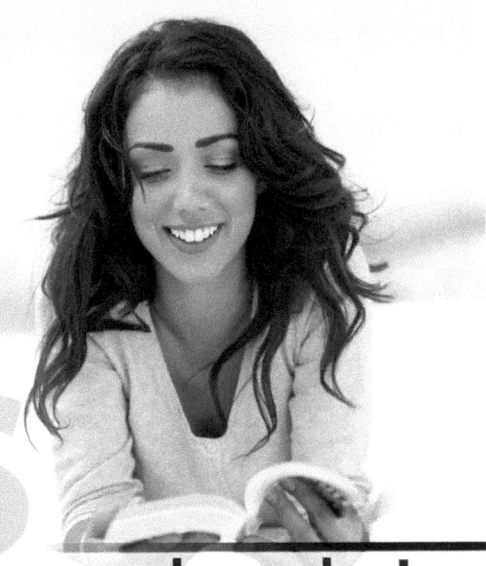
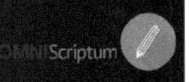

Printed by Books on Demand GmbH, Norderstedt / Germany